Health
and the
Horoscope

Helen Adams Garrett

ISBN-10: 0-86690-624-X
ISBN-13: 978-0-86690-624-1

Cover Design: Jack Cipolla

Published by:
American Federation of Astrologers, Inc.
6535 S. Rural Road
Tempe AZ 85283

www.astrologers.com

Printed in the United States of America

Dedication

This work is dedicated to those who
devote their time and talents to natural
and nutritional health and healing,
and to researchers of medical astrology
and metaphysics.

Contents

Introduction

The chapters in this book that relate to the appetite and nutrition were originally written in 1986 with my late husband as coauthor. Jim had been ill since before I knew him but we used nutrition to keep him well enough to enjoy astrological conventions and travel. We wanted to share some of what we had learned with people who had the same interest. Since his death I have learned much more and some of the information is included in this book.

His chart is used as the example in the chapter in this book on interpretation and aspects.

It is my personal belief that we cannot add one day to our life span but that we can enhance the quality along the way. It also seems to me that our degree of immunity differs according to our heritage, nutritional habits, geographical location, mental attitude and especially our emotional stability which, when entwined with our mental adjustments, or wellness, adds up to stress.

It is these things that we can control that we will consider here. Many times we are not aware that a choice makes a difference, but scientific studies show that it does.

A year before my husband died he had a serious attack which we turned around with food. His doctor came to his hospital room and sat on the floor for more than an hour asking questions beginning with, "How did you do that?"

What we eat is important. Natural, fresh, succulent and preferably raw is best. It tastes so good and has most of the nutrients we need. We are what we eat, so food is astrology too.

Just before going to the hospital for the last time, Jim looked at an ephemeris and said, "If I can make it until 6:00 am, I may live awhile longer."

I never knew on what he based that statement. Jim died March 28, 1986, 5:50 am, Belleville, Illinois.

Be healthy and be happy.

Chapter 1

Quadruplicity of Physical Ailments

Since we are what we eat, our physical condition, whether in strength or weakness, is reflected in the nature of the signs on the angles, the Sun or Ascendant. The sign of the Moon and the sixth house cusp also reflect the health conditions. There will be more about this later.

It takes the average of too much and too little to equal a normal or ideal diet. Hence, less than half of our health and food behavior is ideal.

Cardinal Signs

In matters of food and health, the cardinal signs—Aries, Cancer, Libra and Capricorn—represent the head, stomach, kidneys and knees, which will be affected to some extent. To illustrate, let us say someone has a severe sinus headache (Aries). Soon he begins to feel nauseous (Cancer), winds up on his knees (Capricorn) over the toilet, and on the first heave, kidney action (Libra) causes urine to flow.

Aries: Aries ailments are of the head or parts of the head from the jaw hinge, including only the upper teeth and upward. This means eyes, sinus problems, facial twitches, upper teeth, ear infections, hair falling out, face flushes, and fevers that cause the face to feel overly heated. It is estimated that more than eighty percent of blind people are also diabetic, a Libra disease; blindness is Aries.

Cancer: Cancer ailments are of the stomach, digestion, emotional disturbances or the breasts of both sexes. The fatality rate of men who get breast cancer is far higher than the rate among women who get breast cancer. People who have cancer and go back to the origin of their disease find that it had an emotional root. For this reason, cancer has high standing in the cardinal signs. Ulcers and digestive problems are also high-risk ailments.

Libra: Libra ailments are of the kidneys, ovaries, and testes. Diabetes and Libra sentimentality relates strongly to diseases of the lymphatic system. One only needs to think back over the illnesses experienced within two years following the loss of a lover, spouse, or various types of love relationships to be able to associate the physical ailment to the partnership quality of the sign Libra. A general feeling of not being loved is a prime contributor to Libra ailments.

Capricorn: Capricorn ailments are of the knees, bones, cartilage, teeth, nails, and any body part supported by calcium. Some illnesses are arthritis, bodily decay as a result of bad teeth, gallstones, osteoporosis, or deterioration caused by prolonged or chronic constipation. One of these illnesses might manifest as a result of loss of respect. Former President Richard M. Nixon, a Capricorn, had phlebitis.

Aries

If the Sun, Moon or Ascendant is in Aries, Mars is in the first house or Aries rules the sixth house, you reflect the Aries/cardinal reaction in matters of food and health.

The natural taste desire of Aries is hot and spicy. Highly seasoned foods appeal to the appetite. This includes the nitrates, which are sharp in taste. Aries eats fast and does not mind eating

2

alone. Zesty hors d'oeuvres and bite-size things are favorites for this category.

The danger for the Aries/cardinal appetite is that spices and strong seasonings must stay on the move in the body to be beneficial. If they lag in the system, the individual can develop ulcers, sediments in the kidneys or impurities in the blood stream. These contribute to discomfort by way of headache, stomach ache, kidney problems, constipation, or arthritis. Any or all of these could damage the eyes.

The Aries appetite needs an abundance of liquids to keep spices beneficial. When used in proportion, spices are very valuable; but just as an abrasive cleans the kitchen floor, too much of it will destroy the finish. An addition of select carbohydrates can help to absorb the excess spices, but it is best to regulate consumption. One great advantage of spicy foods is they keep the bodily fluids in good circulation and thus assist in protecting the individual from heart problems. They also open the nasal passages for more free and deep breathing. Cayenne pepper is extremely beneficial to blood circulation, opening sinuses and reducing high blood pressure.

Conflicting energy of the four cardinal signs manifests ill health unless we capitalize on handicaps. On the other hand, if we moderate food intake in balance with the body's needs, health is greatly improved. Hot and spicy foods, representative of Aries, stimulate blood flow, enhancing better heart function relative to the sign of Leo and purification of the blood as relative to the third fire sign, Sagittarius.

Cancer

If the Sun, Moon or Ascendant is in Cancer, the Moon is in the first house or Cancer is on the sixth house cusp, you reflect the cardinal reaction in matters of food and health.

The natural taste desire of Cancer is for carbohydrates (starch). Sugars are starches but sweets are not necessarily nor expressly the desired taste of Cancer. Basic carbohydrates are gravy, pasta, bread, pie, cake, and cereal, the major ingredients in this example being the grains. Then there are the starchy vegetables such as beans, peas, potatoes, and corn. An alternative to yeast as a leavening agent for bread is baking powder, which has a very high aluminum content. It is now known that aluminum is the predominant element responsible for Alzheimer's disease. Knowing this, along with the fact that Cancer-type people are often moody (Moon-ruled), allows us to better understand why.

Carbohydrates prevent hunger. This is the reason bread is known as the staff of life, but most modern day bread cannot support life in a healthy manner because the flour has been stripped of its value to give it longer shelf life. This means the natural vitamins have been removed and chemistry has been added. Many of the whole grain breads on store shelves today are about half white (chloride bleached) flour, and even the whole grain has been stripped of the portion of the grain that causes it to sprout new plants. That part of the grain is the germ or Vitamin E, and the reason why most Americans should take about 200 units of Vitamin E every day.

Most pasta is made from refined (stripped) flour. Anyone depending on a pasta diet to take off weight will be unsuccessful if eating refined pasta with a cream sauce made of refined thickeners, high fat and sugar, which most commercial and restaurant sauces contain abundantly. The beautifully sculptured women who stay beautiful on pasta are Italian and do not use refined ingredients or canned sauce. Trim Italian families use truly natural foods. Be aware that refined carbohydrates are stripped of their food value and thus add poundage. Most victims claim they don't eat that much, which is probably true, but one tablespoon of ketchup is twenty-nine percent sugar, whereas the same amount of chocolate ice cream contains only twenty-one percent sugar. A hefty blob of ketchup will add more weight than the hamburger you dash it on because you burn the calories of the meat, which is not the case with sugar in ketchup.

Rice also deserves a few words. Rice is a marvelously healthy food when in its complete state, known as brown rice. White rice is pretty but it has only empty calories that add weight. Empty calories add weight by absorbing and holding fluids; they do not supply energy. So the people who do not acknowledge the danger of refined carbohydrates just keep eating refined foods and sit and sit and sit while they gain more and more and more unsightly pounds.

The danger of the Cancer appetite is in becoming overweight, suffering from diabetes, kidney problems, headaches (resulting from lack of circulation), overindulgence (connected with emotional stress, which can result in ulcers or cancer) and intestinal concrete, otherwise identified as constipation. It is wise to follow the appetite needs, not the appetite urges.

The Cancer appetite needs bulk to eliminate hunger pangs and fiber to keep the food on the move and improve metabolism. The answer is natural; it gives a clear head to Aries, dietary satisfaction to Cancer, beautiful bodies to Libra, and healthy endurance to Capricorn.

Libra

If the Sun, Moon, or Ascendant is in Libra, Venus is in the first house or Libra is the sign on the sixth house cusp, you reflect the cardinal reaction (Libra, Capricorn, Aries, Cancer) in matters of food and health.

The natural taste desire of Libra is for the mildly sweet and beautiful. Food must have eye appeal. Salads and desserts are the pretty dishes, and the actual serving dish is also important to the food enjoyment of a Libra. It is not unusual for the Libra food influence to forego an entire meal in exchange for a dessert, rationalizing that a meal with dessert is excessive and a dessert alone is acceptable.

The instinct is to arrange the food artistically and colorfully on the plate. A little bite of everything is more exciting than an indulgence in one or two items. For the precise taste preference, ask every Libra-influenced person you know to tell you what their favorite food or taste is, and you will be amazed at the variety of replies you get. Generally, hard raw food will not be the favorite. They make too much noise to chew. The greasy look is unappealing, casting out the fat appearance of some meats. But they go big time for cream sauces, which have thousands of hidden calories. The fluffy look attracts the Libra appetite.

I know a lovely lady who is a Libra type, and when she attends a share-a-dish-dinner she always takes a pink cake with a fluffy icing. She buys the cake already baked and iced. The Libra type would rather set a pretty table than cook a meal. Salad is another good job assignment for them.

The danger for Libra is in developing an inability to process carbohydrates that convert to sugar, and other sugars, resulting in a disposition toward diabetes. Another danger is the collection of sediment in the kidneys. Libra, being beauty conscious, might experiment with extreme weight loss diets for short periods of time; however, they tend to revert to the old routine of regular and irregular diets, depending on their social schedule and partnerships.

The Libra appetite needs liquids to flush the kidneys and lean protein for strength because the delicacy of Libra has a strong mental constitution but not an abundance of muscle power.

Capricorn

If the Sun, Moon or Ascendant is in Capricorn, Saturn is in the first house or Capricorn is the sign on the sixth house cusp, you reflect the Capricorn/cardinal reaction in matters of food and health.

The natural taste desire of Capricorn is for lean meat and high protein vegetables. Some favorites are peanut butter, cooked vegetables, and non-fattening foods in general. Convenience is a key word. Casserole dishes were most certainly originated by Capricorn. It is a very wise, appealing, tasty and economical production, provided the contents are not toxic from holding too long.

Capricorn's danger is infrequent "grease jobs and oil changes." Olive oil, which is a lubricant, might be an advantage, and the same is true of celery, celery juice, and apple cider vinegar. These are solvents that can dissolve and wash away excess mineral collections.

Capricorn has a high intake of minerals and low intake of natural lubricating materials. This condition does not allow calcium to be properly assimilated, and calcium deposits can occur in the joints or even close to internal organs as gall or kidney stones, interfering with the organ's function.

Capricorn needs more raw fruit and vegetables for intestinal cleansing, along with proper physical exercise to assimilate calcium. Capricorn also needs to move around while working rather than continuously staying in one spot.

The conflicting cardinal energy develops in granular deposits in the joints, especially in and around the knees. It is extraordinarily important that the Capricorn type keep moving. Mild exercise, even in the form of walking, is of ultimate importance to Capricorn. Exercise is the only thing that will prevent some kinds of joint disorders. Surgery is not the answer because even doctors admit that if it helps, it is only a small amount. Walking will absorb the misplaced calcium and actually heal the offenders.

What else will walking do? It will keep the Aries energy happy because of movement. It aids digestion for the Cancer energy and it makes the Libra energy stay young and beautiful.

Capricorn is of the earth element; consequently the addition of fruit and vegetables to the diet pleases the Virgo needs in the Capricorn-influenced chart because it tends to settle anxieties. The proper Capricorn intake of food will allow the Taurus area of the individual to be able to relax and perform responsibilities more easily, promptly and accurately, all being appropriate to the satisfaction of Capricorn.

Fixed Signs

The fixed signs are Taurus, Leo, Scorpio, and Aquarius. The word "fixed" describes the directive energy of these signs. There are a few words that are, perhaps, more explanatory than fixed, such as strong-willed, persistent, persevering, and enduring. This lets us know right away that these are the signs that will experience ill health related to stress (Taurus), exhaustion from control efforts (Leo), fear of the unknown (Scorpio), and fatigue and pressure (Aquarius).

High blood pressure is directly related to heart problems, stroke, accidents, and general frustration. The quadruplicate cycle is that of building. Taurus is the worker who needs to rest, Leo the royal overseer who gets heart trouble when things go wrong, Scorpio strains a muscle, and Aquarius gets strung out over the self-imposed requirement of having to stay with a project. A fixed reaction illness will usually announce its presence following a chronic symptom or condition.

Taurus: Taurus ailments frequently have their origin in the throat and are closely related to the thyroid and the ability or inability to relax. A healthy Taurus-type person is always willing to work for value or fair pay. This is the sign of the highest pain tolerance of the zodiac, but Libra, the other Venus-ruled sign, runs a close second. A Taurus-dominant person who cannot be motivated and is always thought of as lazy has an organic malfunction. It is time for thyroid and metabolic testing.

Leo: Leo ailments relate to the heart and the spine. Their discomforts come when self-esteem is lowered if the individual is unable to keep control of what he considers his small-world empire. It might be a result of a romantic upset, which is one of the major factors of suicide in teenagers, and results from a feeling of defeat or failure. When a Leo-type person labors under these deterrents of seif-esteem, it is difficult to stand tall and the spine begins to crumble and bend.

8

Scorpio: Scorpio ailments relate to the reproductive organs, the elimination systems, and muscles. Too little or too much, one way or another, can be abusive for the reproductive organs. Holding on to deep emotions and long-term resentment are the contributing factors. The elimination area covers the bladder, hemorrhoids, and sinuses. Sinus pain and infection are Aries-related, but the chambers and elimination canals are Scorpio. Under normal conditions, Scorpio is the healthiest sign of the zodiac and is also the strongest per cubic inch of the body. It is never wise for the Scorpio type to delay healing efforts because there is not an abundance of natural antibiotic available since the body only produces it when needed.

Aquarius: The ailments of the Aquarius type are related to circulation and are especially notable in the lower legs, which are the circulatory system's turning point back to the heart. This is the reason why walking is such a valuable movement. It is now believed by many members of the medica! profession that walking is the most complete and most perfect cure for circulation blockages, even over surgery or medication, if not neglected too long. Circulation of the body fluids, which take antibodies and white blood cells to any part of the body that is ailing is an Aquarius assignment. Circulation into and out of society also strongly affects Aquarius types. Restrictions that prevent open expression of individuality are very upsetting to Aquarius energy. The results contribute to strokes and nerve diseases, which come from the spine, such as Parkinson's disease and palsy.

Taurus

If the Sun, Moon or Ascendant is in Taurus, Venus is in the first house or Taurus rules the sixth house, you reflect the fixed/reaction in matters of food and health. Your strengths and weaknesses affect the throat, physical energy, heart, spine, body elimination capabilities, reproductive organs, nerve fluids involving motivation of energy and circulation of fluids that take antibodies to any part of the body that requires healing.

The natural taste desires of Taurus are for beef and protein, chocolate in some form and good food in general. Taurus is a connoisseur of food. The quality of Taurus has the best taste buds of the zodiac. The taste choices are for foods that determine strength accompanied by an ability to relax. Taurus likes stable meals with good desserts, which probably contributes to a tendency toward excess weight after middle age.

The danger for the Taurus/fixed appetite is in overeating because of a taste for food that requires rest after eating. Taurus need always to remember that in order to keep weight at a proper level it is essential not to eat more food than can be utilized. Of course that is the trap. When Taurus works, Taurus works, and eating can be postponed. When Taurus plays, Taurus plays, thereby using energy. When Taurus is doing nothing, Taurus is not really doing nothing; Taurus is eating. Then one day the stark realization dawns that it is easier and more fun to put weight on than to take it off.

The Taurus appetite needs physical exercise in order to balance the food intake and should generally reduce desserts to half portions for the most benefit. Sufficient protein is usually present in the diet of most Taurus-dominant people provided there is a trim fat habit. The desire for chocolate can become an addiction to them just as other signs can become addicted to various foods. A constant practice of renewing motivation is the one most important recommendation to Taurus-type people.

The conflicting energy of the fixed signs creates stress for Taurus, but the triplicity of the earth signs Virgo and Capricorn enhance the Taurus-dominant person by stimulating the desire to succeed. The Virgo energy encourages Taurus to be practical in food intake and to follow the rules that assist one in feeling good daily. Capricorn helps to effectuate self-discipline; with Taurus, one performance is an experience, a second performance is testimony to having benefitted from the first experience, and the third performance becomes a well-formed habit that Taurus fully believes has always been in effect.

Leo

If the Sun, Moon or Ascendant is in Leo, the Sun is in the first house or Leo is the sign on the sixth house cusp, you reflect the fixed reaction in matters of food and health.

The natural taste desire of the Leo type is for rich, regal, elegant foods, as well as display and impression. Many times Leo wilt order the most expensive steak on the menu, eat only a few bites, and leave the remainder to be cast out with the kitchen garbage. It would not be a regal act to take home a leftover, but the impression of "the best" has been made. Better quality meat of course has marbled fat, and for Leo it is more beneficial to toss it rather than add more cholesterol to already over-packed blood vessels. Among the favorites are rich cream sauces, salad dressings and dips with high fat content enhanced with sugar, and desserts made with real butter, cream, sugar, and eggs, and then piled high with whipped cream or decorative icing made with more butter or cream.

The danger for the Leo fixed appetite is the intake of excessive food which leaves unfriendly cholesterol in the system. Emotional stress in love relationships lowers self-esteem, sometimes promoting compulsive eating and, thus, overindulgence. Then depression begins. Leo types tend to lose their hair when things go askew, and this would imply a chemical imbalance possibly due to excessive fat and rich foods.

The Leo appetite needs to be more aware of the energy from omega-3, certain fish oils, and the value of vegetable oils over damages caused by animal fat. It is wise to choose high protein, low-fat meat. Practically all berries are blood cleansers, and grapes are exceptionally good. The emotional balance can evolve in becoming aware of pleasures that other people stimulate as opposed to repelling others by being too focused on oneself. Sincere compliments accumulate tremendous returns in the Leo type.

Conflicting energy from the negative side of Scorpio can cause the Leo to be unhappy by holding resentment. These feelings usually arise out of romantic or professional jealousies. Starvation might be the outlet that endeavors to offset the unwanted emotion. Being bored by uninteresting social deadwood can cause a drain of the proud Leo energy. Professional competition for the dollar would be the last arm of the windmill.

Drawing on the triplicity of the fire element can be supportive. Sagittarius is outgoing and optimistic, and incorporating these positive expressions might be inspirational. Foods of the Sagittarius quality promote good energy without fat, and the positive diet of Sagittarius also includes blood builders.

Scorpio

If the Sun, Moon, or Ascendant is in Scorpio, Pluto is in the first house or Scorpio is the sign on the sixth house cusp, you reflect the fixed reaction in matters of food and health. Your strengths and weaknesses affect the channels of elimination and circulatory and reproductive and metabolic systems.

The natural taste desire of Scorpio is an extremely high protein diet accompanied by a feeling of deprivation if many hours go by without substantial protein. Protein builds muscles and promotes sex drive, the reason why most vegetarians are more or less of the take it or leave it category when it comes to sexual activity. Remember, this is the healthy sign, perhaps because of the attraction to wholesome, simple food rather than junk food.

The danger of the Scorpio/fixed sign is in holding toxins and intestinal gas as a result of excessive animal fat. The byproducts of protein do not eliminate quickly from the body. Hemorrhoids can result from the absence of fiber foods, and there can be odor from gas and sweat glands. Pluto and Scorpio rule odors and will be found in adverse aspect or placement when one experiences unpleasant body odors. The marked determination of Scorpio brings stress on the heart, the back, and energy levels.

Scorpio's diet usually needs more concentration on diaphoretic and spices to stimulate perspiration. Cayenne pepper is a great spice and mango is a leading solid food to help combat any ailment that could benefit from "sweating it out of your system."

Aquarius

If the Sun, Moon or Ascendant is in Aquarius, Uranus is in the first house, or Aquarius is on the cusp of the sixth house, you reflect the fixed/reaction in matters of food and health.

Strengths and weaknesses affect the higher plane nervous system and intellectuality. Aquarius must have certain freedoms or suffer in general motivation, energy output, heart action, or sexual participation.

The natural taste desire of Aquarius is for the unusual. It may take the form of a casserole, bologna, pizza, hot pepper cheese rolled in nuts, peanut butter and honey cookies or a wild duck stuffed with chestnuts and oysters. Eating on routine is not in the vocabulary of the Aquarius type. They starve to the point of nibbling a feast just prior to the main meal and then not a bite when the meal is served.

The danger for Aquarius is in the acid/alkaline balance in the body, which is usually too acid. Lasting energy is in alkaline foods, and the absence of that alkaline energy demands something be eaten immediately. One of the first symptoms to being too acid is tooth tartar. All meat is acid. Most carbohydrates, some dried beans, peas, pasta, rice, and cheese convert to acid immediately upon blending with saliva. In order to be healthy there must be a balance between acid and alkaline. Alkaline foods are all fresh fruit and vegetables. A very efficient way to balance acid and alkaline is to eat something from both lists at each meal and, when in doubt, drink a glass of water with about one-half teaspoon apple vinegar in it now and again. This suggestion for acid/alkaline balance is not just for the Aquarius, but for all signs and anyone who has tartar collect on the teeth.

Most signs and reaction groups need more water and more fiber. Aquarius usually needs a reduction of protein and more starches and vitamins found in fruit and fresh vegetables. The nervous condition of Aquarius is out of sorts if forced to eat on a schedule rather than on a whim.

Mutable Signs

The strengths and weaknesses of the mutable signs—Gemini, Virgo, Sagittarius, Pisces—in food and health are the respiratory system, intestines, blood, thighs, feet, and membranes that form mucus. Even though Gemini is the only mental element included in this list, all of these signs are mental to a great degree. Let's follow them through. Gemini reads something and gets a terrific idea, the idea needs perfection and order (Virgo), suddenly it grows out of perspective and blows the budget (Sagittarius), and ends up with a mental health prescription (Pisces).

Gemini: Gemini ailments are of the respiratory system, arms and hands, shoulders, and the nervous system. Pneumonia is strong on this list. Injured hands, fingers, and arms also get a goodly amount of attention. Muscle strains of the arms and shoulders can be frequent.

Virgo: Virgo ailments usually relate to the intestines. Another potential ailment for Virgo is a lack of muscular development due to the minimal intake of protein. They are the natural vegetarians. The clean crisp way of life appeals to Virgo. Appendicitis is a Virgo malady, and Virgo types also become host to parasites.

Sagittarius: Sagittarius ailments can usually be identified by a blood test, and the chances are that there will be too much of something. The tendency is to diseases that affect the lower extremities or to injuries to that part of the body. Such injuries could well be from sports activities or horseback riding. Discomfort in the hip and lower spine also belong to Sagittarius. A high percentage of elderly die from complications of broken hip injuries.

Pisces: Pisces ailments tend strongly toward collection of mucus. These ailments can be in most any part of the body. Perhaps this is why the soles of the feet, ruled by Pisces, reflect every disor-

14

der of the body. Mucus collects in the respiratory tract, bowels, throat, membranes separating the reproductive organs, sinuses, and in many other remote places. When mucus forms we know something needs attention. We might say that part of the body is requesting sympathy.

Gemini

If the Sun, Moon, or Ascendant is in Gemini, Mercury is in the first house or Gemini is on the sixth house cusp, you reflect the mutable/reaction in the matters of food and health. The Gemini strengths and weaknesses are found in the lungs, nervous system, intestinal tract, blood, or ailments relating to mucus and infection.

The natural taste desire of Gemini is guided by mental attitude of what is it, where did it come from and is it safe? Gemini favorites can be held in the hand—cookies, finger foods, sandwiches, nuts, chips, cheese and crackers, fruits, etc. Gemini likes to eat and read, eat and ride, eat and play games, eat and anything—two things at a time.

Gemini, as a rule, is not strongly attracted to sweets and fatty foods. However, over the past twenty-five years I have seen a lot of overweight Gemini Sun people. I believe the explanation is because of two things: high calorie fried fat on chips and tacos and high calorie fat in cream sauces, fast food, and salad dressing. Gemini eats on the run; fast food places allow for that.

The danger for the Gemini/mutable appetite is that too many foods that are portable do not supply the vitamins and minerals found in vegetables and blood-cleansing fruit. Gemini eats to live and is often known to forget to eat if it is not convenient. Nervous energy requires as many calories as physical exertion.

Gemini needs calming foods such as oatmeal, cabbage, lettuce (a sedative), corn, turkey, and chamomile tea. A major necessity for Gemini is to remember to wind down before going to bed in order to get restful sleep. Avoiding sodas and caffeine is advisable for Gemini.

The conflicting energy of Virgo is often stressful to Gemini because of the nitty-gritty details. Although Gemini loves cars, telephones, and play land rides, long distance trips vital to Sagittarius are not as appealing because Gemini is adaptable to the immediate community where the knowledge of shopping places is no object. Gemini knows what Gemini knows and the life of mystery projected by Pisces energy is confusing to Gemini. Gemini is like a butterfly without a petal to perch on when too heavily exposed to the mutable quadruplicity of Virgo, Sagittarius, Pisces, and Gemini. The mental signs of Libra and Aquarius are more soothing and challenging to Gemini, encouraging the relaxation that promotes better health.

Virgo

If the Sun, Moon, or Ascendant are in Virgo, Mercury is in the first house, or if Virgo is on the sixth house cusp, you reflect the flexible or mutable/reaction in the matters of food and health. Your strengths and weaknesses affect the intestines, conditions of the blood, pockets of mucus, and personal expression through the respiratory system and actual means and methods of communication.

The natural taste desire of Virgo is for vegetables, including grains, which are good for the digestive tract by supplying sufficient enzymes. Cleanliness is a must, but it is difficult to remove all impurities from raw foods, especially with the economical preservation methods used in food in the United States. Also, parasites target raw food persons. Virgo prefers to keep foods separated and simple in recipes. Casseroles with mixed ingredients are not appealing unless every piece of vegetable and meat is truly visible and distinguishable.

The danger for the Virgo/flexible appetite is a shortage of energy and muscle-building foods. Muscles need not be of the demonstrative sports type to be useful. Even the light weight of a writing pen requires muscle movement and the rapid movement of fingers on a keyboard requires even more muscles. The Virgo natural taste sometimes gets out of balance nutritionally when too little meat protein is consumed.

Protein is necessary to help protect the body against disease. Virgos are sensitive to the body when its energy is low, and they tend to vocally acknowledge their symptoms. Consequently, Virgo is recognized as one who tends to be a hypochondriac or at least a chronic complainer.

Virgo needs ample protein, not fat. There is protein in low-fat meat byproducts, but it's wise to consult the label on cheese for fat content because it can vary considerably. Nuts, whole grains, especially brown rice and legumes, including beans of all kinds, peanuts being one, are all high in vegetable protein.

The exactness of Virgo is somewhat aggravated by the carelessness of Sagittarius, the nonchalance of Pisces and the know-it-all attitude of Gemini, all of which contribute to emotional frustration and thus produce bouts of diarrhea, which are frequently experienced by Virgo types. This quadruplicity is highly nervous. The triplicity of the element earth, of which Virgo is one, is calming to Virgo, but these Taurus and Capricorn energies can give rise to plotting and planning. All of the above are in keeping with the Virgo eating routine, which often results in repetitive eating habits that deny foods with a sufficient variety of nourishment.

Sagittarius

If the Sun, Moon, or Ascendant is in Sagittarius, Jupiter is in the first house, or Sagittarius is on the sixth house cusp, you tend to reflect the flexible/reaction in food and health.

Your strengths and weaknesses affect your spiritual attitude and your good luck; physically, you are subject to blood disorders, mobility of the lower limbs, mucus buildup, adverse respiratory conditions, and abnormal intestinal actions.

The natural taste desires of Sagittarius vary and are adventurous. "All you can eat" is an appealing invitation. Meals might be skipped for a day or more, then one to three are eaten. Sometimes even four different orders are consumed in one sitting. Sagittarius always has some favorite taste listed on an exotic menu.

The danger for the Sagittarius/flexible appetite is in overworking the liver by eating too little, then too much. Involuntary body functions operate all the time, and when there is a long period of idleness in the diet, malfunctions tend to occur.

Sagittarius needs more routine in the diet and usually more guidance in what to eat. But then who can guide a Sagittarian attitude into or out of anything?

This freedom-loving sign is self-confident and does not seek Pisces faith. Sagittarius is too high-minded to be grounded by the simplicity of Gemini, and is fully bored by the precision of Virgo. Be grateful for the fire triplicity and the complementary energy of Aries and Leo, which are exciting to Sagittarius. Aries allows Sagittarius to eat at will and Leo enjoys the exotic flamboyance of Sagittarius, each complimenting the other.

Pisces

If the Sun, Moon, or Ascendant is in Pisces, Neptune is in the first house, or if Pisces is on the sixth house cusp, you reflect the flexible/Pisces reaction in matters of food and health.

Your strengths and weaknesses affect your sympathetic system, mucus, respiratory system, intestinal tract, and content and quality of blood. You are sympathetic and compassionate toward less fortunate people to the extent that you may telepathically transmit their ailments to yourself. You are a trap for toxins by way of your lungs, intestines, and blood. It is extremely important for you to detoxify regularly. Colds are still a mystery to the medical profession, possibly because they refuse to accept the fact that colds seem to appear in direct relationship to emotional upsets, and they tend to immediately follow within two to three days of the upset. Colds produce mucus. Pisces is emotional and, although inclined to complain, often won't do so about the current issue that was the cause of the upset. In fact, the cause of the emotional pain could have occurred years prior, yet have only recently been renewed.

The natural taste desire of Pisces is for rich, moist and wet food and for tender protein, such as fish and seafood. Sauces on vegetables, toast, or meat appeal to you. Favorites are fish and meat soups and stews with big beautiful chunks of your choice of vegetables. Meat with gravy and fluffy potatoes draw your attention.

The danger for the Pisces/flexible or mutable appetite is in subsidizing mucus. You are generally attracted to milk and grain foods, both of which are congestive and tend to encourage phlegm and mucus. These should be limited or totally avoided when one has a cold or is experiencing a respiratory attack. Another danger for Pisces types is the sympathetic system, which leads to excessive alcohol intake.

Pisces needs expectorants, something to release phlegm from the throat and bronchial tubes, and antitoxins. Coconut, green leafy vegetables, carrots, garlic, coarse grain, fruits, cayenne pepper, and other readily available suggestions in tablet or capsule form in the health food stores might prove highly beneficial. An old remedy for weaning one from medication or alcohol is cayenne pepper in hot liquids, tea, soup, or vegetable broth.

It is easy to see the conflict with the other mutable signs. Gemini foods are portable, and soup likes to sit on the table. Virgo's fresh, crisp fruit and vegetables are not soft and cuddly in the mouth. Sagittarius' now and then necessary meals are not sufficient for indulgent Pisces. It is certainly easy to understand the compatibility of food and health with the signs of the water triplicity. Cancer serves food or cooks, hot, cool, dry or wet. What one does in the presence of Scorpio gets an indifferent acceptance so long as it does not interfere.

Chapter 2

Dignities and Debilities

Planet and Sign Relationships

Dignity means the planet is in its own sign. Detriment means a planet is in the sign opposing the sign it rules. Exaltation means a planet is in a sign where it is comfortable. Fall means a planet is in the sign opposing exaltation, and thus uncomfortable.

Sun

Dignified in Leo	Exalted in Aries
Detriment in Aquarius	Fall in Libra

The Sun is accidentally dignified in the fifth house, Leo's natural place, and whenever it is in the sign it rules, Leo.

The Sun is at detriment in the opposing sign of Aquarius, which does not seek the limelight and whose priorities are in working out solutions for mankind rather than for self. Aquarius can be embarrassed by excessive attention.

The Sun is exalted in Aries. It is comfortable there. Aries accepts help that the Sun supplies.

The Sun is at fall in Libra, the sign opposing Aries. Libra does not desire to be the focal point but wishes to share position.

Without the authority of the Sun there would be no light or vitality. When the Sun rises, it gets attention and when it doesn't (or when it sets) it is missed, as is any good executive. The Sun has great influence and importance and appears proud. The Sun rules Leo and the Leo keywords are interchangeable.

To interpret the Sun in any other sign, give it the kind of authority described by the sign:

- *Sun in Aries:* self-authority; do own thing
- *Sun in Taurus:* authority over possessions
- *Sun in Gemini:* authority on general information
- *Sun in Cancer:* authority over family and home
- *Sun in Leo:* authority over ambition and leadership
- *Sun in Virgo:* authority over health and correctness
- *Sun in Libra:* authority on diplomacy
- *Sun in Scorpio:* authority on regeneration
- *Sun in Sagittarius:* authority on philosophy
- *Sun in Capricorn*: authority over production
- *Sun in Aquarius*: authority on originality
- *Sun in Pisces*: authority on the mysterious

If the power of the Sun or Leo is negatively used, it results in arrogance, conceit, embarrassment, bragging, or haughtiness.

Moon

Dignified in Cancer   Exalted in Taurus

Detriment in Capricorn   Fall in Scorpio

The Moon is accidentally dignified in the fourth house, Cancer's natural place.

The Moon is at detriment in the opposing sign of Capricorn, which is stable and does not like change.

The Moon is exalted in Taurus because Taurus enjoys comforts of home, family, and good food.

22

The Moon is at fall in Scorpio, the sign opposing Taurus, because it is fixed by nature and emotions are hidden and deep, preferring little expression.

The Moon is only seen when it is in position to reflect the Sun's light. The Moon's qualities are useless unless another person reflects a need and will accept nurturing. The Moon describes emotions according to the sign it occupies. Keywords for Cancer and the Moon are interchangeable. To interpret the Moon in any other sign, give it the kind of emotions described by that sign:

- *Moon in Aries:* personal nurturing
- *Moon in Taurus:* nurtures possessions
- *Moon in Gemini:* nurtures knowledge
- *Moon in Cancer:* nurtures through the home
- *Moon in Leo:* nurtures those who will honor
- *Moon in Virgo:* nurtures perfection in others
- *Moon in Libra:* nurtures companionship
- *Moon in Scorpio:* nurtures secretiveness
- *Moon in Sagittarius:* nurtures optimism
- *Moon in Capricorn:* nurtures success
- *Moon in Aquarius:* nurtures original ideas
- *Moon in Pisces:* nurtures sympathy

The Moon that is not adaptable or is excessively changeable is subject to insanity or fickleness, respectively, both of which are a negative expression of emotion.

Mercury

Dignified in Gemini and Virgo	Exalted in Aquarius
Detriment in Sagittarius and Pisces	Fall in Leo

Mercury is dignified in Gemini and Virgo, and accidentally dignified in the third and sixth houses, these signs' natural houses.

Mercury is at detriment in the opposing signs of Sagittarius and Pisces. The qualities of Mercury reflected through Gemini are at detriment in Sagittarius, and the qualities reflected through Virgo are at detriment in Pisces.

Mercury is exalted in Aquarius, where lightning-speed mental reaction produces creative thinking.

Mercury is at fall in Leo because of the tendency to turn attention inward.

Mercury rules two signs, Gemini and Virgo. It is sometimes difficult to separate that which is applicable to each sign.

Gemini	*Virgo*
Communication	Records of communication Perfection of communication
Knowledge	Knowledge of science, sanitation, and health
Neighborhood	Place of work
Local travel	Perfection
Close kin	Inspection

Mercury describes the method of communication:.

- *Mercury in Aries:* quick thoughts and words
- *Mercury in Taurus:* slow, determined thoughts
- *Mercury in Gemini:* insatiable desire for knowledge
- *Mercury in Cancer:* emotional communication
- *Mercury in Leo:* authoritative communication
- *Mercury in Virgo:* detailed precision
- *Mercury in Libra:* polite
- *Mercury in Scorpio:* profound
- *Mercury in Sagittarius:* far reaching
- *Mercury in Capricorn:* serious
- *Mercury in Aquarius:* unique
- *Mercury in Pisces:* quiet and sympathetic

The negative application is critical and gossipy.

24

Venus

Dignified in Taurus and Libra	Exalted in Pisces
Detriment in Aries and Scorpio	Fall in Virgo

Venus is accidentally dignified in houses two and seven, the natural house placements of Taurus and Libra. Venus is dignified in Taurus and Libra.

Venus is at detriment in the opposing signs, Scorpio and Aries, because Scorpio's passion does not necessarily express tenderness (Venus) and Aries' devotion puts all others second to self.

Venus is exalted in Pisces due to its understanding and sympathy.

Venus is at fall in Virgo because Virgo is impersonal.

Venus is the planet of love and beauty, wealth and comfort. Worldly blessings could be a broad concept of Venus. Applicable keywords of Taurus and Libra are:

- *Venus in Aries:* impetuous in love and wealth Venus in Taurus: devoted
- *Venus in Gemini:* dual in affection and more than one source for wealth
- *Venus in Cancer:* emotional love and family wealth
- *Venus in Leo:* ego and individual wealth
- *Venus in Virgo:* selective love, accountable wealth
- *Venus in Libra:* seeks harmony
- *Venus in Scorpio:* passionate, secretive wealth
- *Venus in Sagittarius:* free love and luck in wealth
- *Venus in Capricorn:* deserved love and earned wealth
- *Venus in Aquarius:* friendly love and wealth from strange sources
- *Venus in Pisces:* idealistic love and mysterious wealth

The negative application of Venus is vain, destitute, lazy, or gaudy.

Mars

Dignified in Taurus and Scorpio   Exalted in Aquarius

Detriment in Virgo and Libra   Fall in Cancer

Mars is accidentally dignified in the first and eighth houses, which are the natural places of Aries and Scorpio. Mars is at home and dignified in Aries and Scorpio.

Mars is at detriment in the opposing signs of Libra and Taurus, both being Venus-ruled and of slow nature not readily accepting impulsiveness.

Mars is exalted in Capricorn, where the energy is appreciated for endurance.

Mars is at fall in Cancer, where fire makes steam.

Mars, god of war, represents energy, both physically and passionately, and consequently governs Aries and Scorpio. Aries energy relates more to the individual and oneness, while Scorpio energy relates to that which encompasses others. Insurance, for example, is a pooling of funds, and two people are involved in sex.

Key words of Aries and Scorpio are applicable to Mars by classifying birth and beginnings to the openness and fire of Aries, and by classifying endings, terminations, and deep emotions to Scorpio.

- *Mars in Aries:* aggressive
- *Mars in Taurus:* quieted and slowed down
- *Mars in Gemini:* talkative
- *Mars in Cancer:* emotional
- *Mars in Leo:* ambitious
- *Mars in Virgo:* active in critique
- *Mars in Libra:* argumentative
- *Mars in Scorpio:* forcefully intent
- *Mars in Sagittarius:* a sportsman
- *Mars in Capricorn:* business-like

- *Mars in Aquarius:* socially active
- *Mars in Pisces:* artistic

Negative Mars in physical and personal action promotes accidents; in sexual energy, it promotes perversion.

Jupiter

Dignified in Sagittarius	Exalted in Cancer
Detriment in Gemini	Fall in Capricorn

Jupiter is accidentally dignified in the ninth house, the natural place of Sagittarius. Jupiter is dignified in Sagittarius, which it rules.

Jupiter is at detriment in the opposing sign, Gemini, because Gemini prefers a little knowledge on everything, where Jupiter prefers expansion to specialization.

Jupiter is exalted in Cancer, where it can adapt to "flow with the tide."

Jupiter is at fall in Capricorn because Capricorn is cautious and curbs Jupiter's confidence.

Jupiter is the largest of the planets in our solar system and represents generosity and massiveness. Surrounded by many moons and much gas, Jupiter is capable of expansion in its allotted area. Jupiter can grant many blessings. Its great virtue is optimistic humor.

Jupiter describes its abundance according to the sign of its placement.

- *Jupiter in Aries:* personal promotion
- *Jupiter in Taurus:* expansion of possessions
- *Jupiter in Gemini:* much knowledge
- *Jupiter in Cancer:* fine home, educated family
- *Jupiter in Leo:* fortune and prominence
- *Jupiter in Virgo:* scientific

- *Jupiter in Libra:* legal justice
- *Jupiter in Scorpio:* resourceful
- *Jupiter in Sagittarius:* business success
- *Jupiter in Capricorn:* many friends
- *Jupiter in Aquarius:* spirituality
- *Jupiter in Pisces:* unbelievably imaginative

Negative application of Jupiter can result in selfishness, embezzlement, obesity, carelessness, gluttony, and violation of laws.

Saturn

Dignified in Capricorn   Exalted in Libra

Detriment in Cancer   Fall in Aries

Saturn is accidentally dignified in the tenth house, Capricorn's natural place.

Saturn is dignified in Capricorn, where it is at home.

Saturn is at detriment in the opposing sign, Cancer, because Saturn is stable and Cancer is changeable.

Saturn is exalted in Libra because time for deliberation equals the caution of Saturn in some respects.

Saturn is at fall in Aries because Aries is the sprinter and does not welcome the plodding of Saturn.

Saturn is surrounded by ice rings and so characterizes solidarity. Saturn is old in mythology and has endured. It rules Capricorn, the sign of tradition and the builder of character and reputation.

Applicable keywords that best describe Saturn in the various signs are:

- *Saturn in Aries:* self-discipline
- *Saturn in Taurus:* using material values
- *Saturn in Gemini:* disciplined study
- *Saturn in Cancer:* responsible to family

- *Saturn in Leo:* restricted by authority
- *Saturn in Virgo:* restricted by health
- *Saturn in Libra:* responsibility through partner
- *Saturn in Scorpio:* traditional moral code
- *Saturn in Sagittarius:* philosophical responsibilities
- *Saturn in Capricorn:* rigid training
- *Saturn in Aquarius:* learns by experience
- *Saturn in Pisces:* divine discipline

Saturn also represents denial, usually due to the individual's acceptance of some situations. This attitude promotes negativity because Saturn uses the obstacle as an excuse for failure.

Uranus

Dignified in Aquarius   Exalted in Scorpio

Detriment in Leo   Fall in Taurus

Uranus is accidentally dignified in the eleventh house, which is the natural place of Aquarius. Uranus is dignified in Aquarius, where it is at home.

Uranus is at detriment in the opposing sign of Leo. Uranus looks to the masses, and Leo prefers to be looked upon and recognized.

Uranus is exalted in Scorpio, probably because Scorpio quietly and calmly works out solutions without involving others in conversation concerning the issue. In many ways that is the nature of the sign of Aquarius. Aquarius solves the problem before it is mentioned as a problem.

Uranus is at fall in Taurus because Uranian restlessness is not compatible with Taurean patience.

Representing all that is new and exciting, Uranus rather suddenly came into view of Earth in recent times. The ancients were aware of the influence of Neptune and Pluto, but Uranus came as a surprise, typical of its nature. Uranus shares rulership of Aquarius

29

with Saturn, which explains why some of its qualities do not fit with Saturn.

- *Uranus in Aries:* unique in singularity
- *Uranus in Taurus:* individualistic comforts
- *Uranus in Gemini:* inventive ideas
- *Uranus in Cancer:* modern home
- *Uranus in Leo:* reformation of ego
- *Uranus in Virgo:* scientific revolution
- *Uranus in Libra:* freedom in partnership
- *Uranus in Scorpio:* sexual and moral freedom
- *Uranus in Sagittarius:* specialized expansions
- *Uranus in Capricorn:* unusual business
- *Uranus in Aquarius:* freedom for identity
- *Uranus in Pisces:* individualistic beliefs

There is a fine line between genius and insanity. When Uranian ability is negatively applied, it can become destructive or eccentric.

Neptune

Dignified in Pisces   Exalted in Sagittarius

Detriment in Virgo   Fall in Gemini

Neptune is accidentally dignified in the twelfth house, the natural place of Pisces. Neptune is dignified in Pisces, the sign it rules, where faith can supply all needs.

Neptune is at detriment in Virgo, where realism is a must.

Not all authorities agree with the exaltation of Neptune. I believe Neptune is exalted in Sagittarius because of the similarity with Pisces and the Jupiter co-rulership. This would mean that Neptune is at fall in Gemini, because Gemini is very outspoken.

Pisces, the sign of two fishes swimming in opposite directions, is ruled by Neptune. Faith supplies protection in the uncertainty of direction. It's a big ocean and fish eyes are always open; they have no eyelids, but they do not see clearly and will bite on anything when hungry.

Keywords that best describe Neptune in the various signs are:

- *Neptune in Aries:* know thyself
- *Neptune in Taurus:* unpolished diamond
- *Neptune in Gemini:* a rose by another name
- *Neptune in Cancer:* unknown address
- *Neptune in Leo:* king of romantic phantom nation.
- *Neptune in Virgo:* drugs and bulldozers; clear it up or clean it out
- *Neptune in Libra:* missing partner
- *Neptune in Scorpio:* unknown lover, anyone will do
- *Neptune in Sagittarius:* blind faith
- *Neptune in Capricorn:* corporate conglomerate
- *Neptune in Aquarius*: invention, what is it?
- *Neptune in Pisces:* let God do it

The highest level is total dependency on higher power. The lowest level is dependency on nothing and resorting to low living.

Pluto

Dignified in Scorpio	Exalted in Aries
Detriment in Taurus	Fall in Libra

Pluto is accidentally dignified in the eighth house, the natural house of Scorpio. Pluto is dignified in Scorpio, the sign it rules.

Pluto is at detriment in Taurus because Pluto removes what Taurus builds.

Pluto is exalted in Aries because Aries is appreciative of the energy and action.

Pluto is at fall in Libra because explosiveness is the reverse nature of Libra.

Pluto arrived just prior to the atomic bomb: great power in a minute package. That's Pluto! It wipes away the old to make way for reconstruction. Close scrutiny may reveal great treasures where the ordinary once stood.

Some astrologers pay little attention to Pluto, but each individual is capable of outstanding power in the house where Pluto is found. Alternatively, the individual does not use the power and becomes the victim of others in that area of life.

Applicable keywords that best describe Pluto in the each of the signs are:

- *Pluto in Aries:* new beginnings on old foundations
- *Pluto in Taurus:* destroyed to rebuild
- *Pluto in Gemini:* explosive knowledge
- *Pluto in Cancer:* indoor plumbing
- *Pluto in Leo:* love 'em and leave 'em
- *Pluto in Virgo:* insecticides poison the food but make it perfect.
- *Pluto in Libra:* revoke the laws
- *Pluto in Scorpio:* transformation and reconstruction
- *Pluto in Sagittarius:* evangelism is space
- *Pluto in Capricorn:* earthquakes
- *Pluto in Aquarius:* universal scramble
- *Pluto in Pisces:* the sea turns over

Pluto in a negative sense uses power to destroy for power's sake. Kidnaping, murder, and rape are negative words.

Houses

The houses of a chart represent the departments of life, and the interpretative information closely coincides with the comparable sign of the zodiac. To clarify:

- The first house is comparable to Aries and defines the self, the first person.

- The second house is comparable to Taurus and defines one's income and material values.
- The third house is comparable to Gemini and defines how one thinks and communicates.
- The fourth house is comparable to Cancer and defines the early family life, home and emotional attitudes.
- The fifth house is comparable to Leo and defines one's romances, children, creative ability and choice of entertainment.
- The sixth house is comparable to Virgo and shows work capabilities and potential tendencies for illnesses.
- The seventh house is comparable to Libra and explains one's relationships, especially with the spouse.
- The eighth house is comparable to Scorpio and describes sexual expression and passionate desires for all things material. It also defines moral and spiritual experiences.
- The ninth house is comparable to Sagittarius and portrays philosophical patterns and generosity. It might be said that the ninth house shows how far one can be expected to go.
- The tenth house is comparable to Capricorn and describes the career and honor of the individual.
- The eleventh house is comparable to Aquarius and describes social life and friends.
- The twelfth house is comparable to Pisces and reveals the subconscious, fears and sorrows.

Chapter 3

Interpretation and Aspects

What interpretation is given when more than two planets are involved in an aspect? What procedure is used? What if the energy of one planet in aspect to another is favorable, while a second is in unfavorable aspect?

There are no new rules. It is the same system that has been used for thousands of years. Consider the nature of the planet, its sign, its house, and its aspect to the first planet in question. Always look at which house the planet rules. Hold in mind these factors.

Use the same process on the next planet in aspect, and keep these factors in mind. If there are more aspects to either of the other planets forming a chain of energy, consider each aspect separately.

Now you have the plot for a story. Forget whether you know the person or anything about the event. Put the story together.

The next step is to line up the revealed energy in the order the aspects occur. Separating aspects point to the past. In a natal chart they represent pre-natal events. Applying aspects are developing, to occur later.

When aspecting a transit to a natal or progressed chart you can stretch the aspect if there are no other intervening aspects, and say, for example, "The Sun will square Mars," even though the degree is too wide to be considered a square at the time.

There may be a separating sextile such as transiting Sun sextile natal Mars, indicating that the individual (Sun) may have become aware of a potential (sextile) for action (Mars). Then you might say, "When the Sun is square your Mars you will feel an urgency to act." The square aspect will soon follow the sextile and you know there has been an opportunity. Now advise action.

Of course, hard or adverse aspects to natal Mars may be reckless or forced, but favorable transiting aspects indicate ease or assistance when the time to act arrives. Additionally, outside help from a sextile or a trine from another planet may relieve the stress of a square.

For the order of the exact degree for closing of aspects, consult the aspectarian in your ephemeris. It is tricky to calculate timing when fast moving planets are being computed. Mercury may be very near to closing an aspect and the Moon may be a few degrees from the aspect it is forming. Which will be there first? The race is on. Consult the aspectarian for the easy and accurate conclusion.

In learning techniques in interpretation, go back to the past in your own chart or someone you know well. Look at a few days, week, months, or a year prior to the event and see what transits were touching your natal chart and what progressions were active. Then look at the actual date of the event to see what aspects were exact. Don't be surprised, if Saturn is involved, to find the aspect separating rather than exact or applying. It is Saturn's nature to be delayed, while Mars events may arrive prematurely.

Errors in interpretation frequently are due to choosing the incorrect keyword. Both romance and children are under the fifth house and one may interpret a pleasant and romantic event that instead develops as a delightful accomplishment of a child.

It would be virtually impossible to set up all the various configurations and combinations for study, but we shall endeavor to state keywords and every pattern appropriate to any set of circumstances that may occur. Practice will then allow one to become fairly proficient in interpretation when planets join forces.

This will be illustrated with an example that might have been "a near-death experience" without memory or visions. Breath was not detectable for several minutes.

The natal chart is like a gun, being what it is only because it is what it is. It can only do what it was made to do. An individual can only be what the natal chart promises. But like a gun, it can be cared for, perfected, and polished into excellence. Progressions are ammunition for coming events. The transits pull the trigger.

Interpretation

In the illustrated tri-wheel chart (page 38) for my late husband Jim, the natal Moon ruling the Ascendant and in the twelfth can be self-damaging. It indicates withdrawal from emotional situations because it is the Moon. Moon in Gemini indicates much thought, and in the twelfth house, words would not be consistently voiced.

Look for a progression to supply the ammunition for the natal potential. Venus is at 16 Aries 46 in the tenth house and is the ruler of the fifth house (Libra on the cusp) and the intercepted sign (Taurus) in the eleventh house. This is a separating aspect, so we immediately know that the action was from the past or has been a long time coming.

Considering the unexpressed natal Gemini Moon as "quiet contemplation," it is feasible that the individual had long dealt with disturbing factors concerning emotional expression (Moon) of love (Venus). Love of whom or what? Mother. Venus is in the tenth house, which is one of the parental houses.

Transiting Uranus retrograde in the sixth house of health is trine the progressed Venus. Uranus indicates some kind of action or desire for freedom to be more of what the individual wants to be. In this instance it meant that the individual wanted to express love

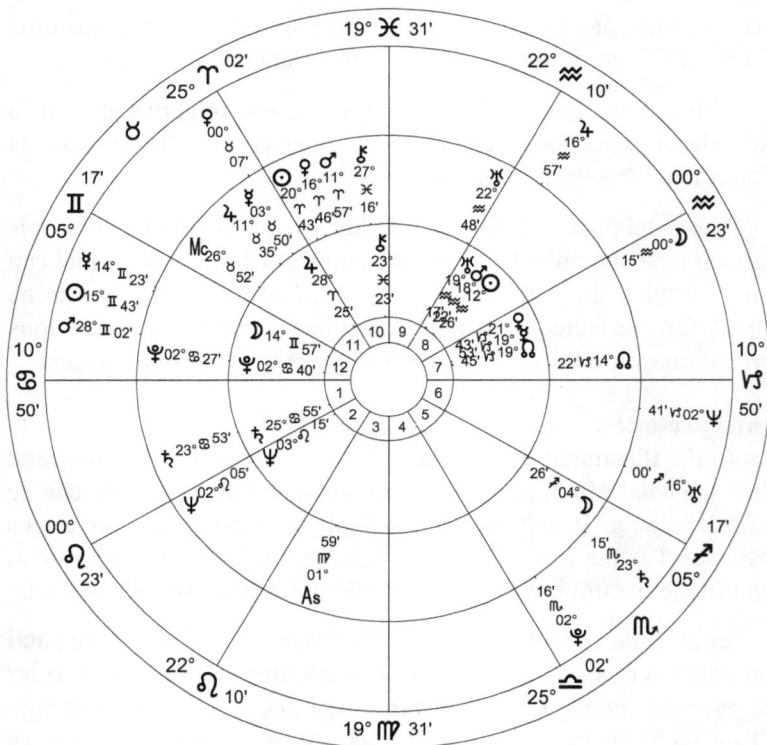

*Jim Garrett. Inner wheel, natal chart; middle wheel, progressed,
June 8, 1985; outer wheel, transits, June 8, 1985*

to the mother in the individual's manner and not in the way the
mother wanted to receive it.

Transiting Uranus is also opposition natal Moon in the sixth/
twelfth polarity. Uranus is the bearer of surprises and the unusual.
It rules the ninth house of the higher mind and is retrograde in the
sixth house of health, so the aspect had just passed. The native had
been ill since January 16, 1985, when Uranus was in close opposition to the natal Moon. At that time, transiting Mars was in Pisces.

38

On January 16 the illness became known. On that date, Jupiter, the sixth house ruler, opposed natal Saturn, and the transiting Sun was conjunct transiting Jupiter and opposing natal Saturn. Transiting Saturn was trine natal Saturn, and the Jupiter-Sun conjunction was sextile transiting Saturn. These aspects were favorable to the outcome, although it would take time.

Let's go back to the natal Moon opposition transiting Uranus. The probability of improving health (sixth house) behind the scenes (twelfth house) through things of the higher mind (Uranus rules the ninth house) had potential.

Progressed Venus was more than a degree past a sextile to natal Moon. This means it is an old problem. Uranus was coming to a trine with the progressed Venus, indicating help. The native had chosen metaphysical and alternative treatment from the beginning in preference to surgery.

On May 14, 1985, when Jupiter was transiting the native's eighth house within minutes of an exact sextile to both progressed Venus and transiting Uranus, the native saw a surgeon because there was a remaining block that had not cleared. Outpatient tests were ordered.

Meanwhile, the patient was improving.

Hospitalization for more tests and impending surgery came on June 5, when the transiting Sun conjoined the natal Moon. The physical condition was greatly improved since the physician had seen the patient, but tests still seemed to be in order. A second physician was consulted, and on June 6, 1985 at 2:30 pm CDT, the native underwent a test of the pancreas. During the test, his breathing temporarily ceased, requiring the emergency use of a respirator.

What happened? Transiting Moon was at 4 Aquarius 16 in the sign of the unexpected, emergencies, the unusual and unplanned, near the native's eighth house cusp. Transiting Mercury (breathing) was conjunct the transiting Sun and natal Moon in the twelfth house. Transiting Jupiter was applying to a sextile to progressed Venus and was sextile transiting Uranus. Jupiter trine natal Moon, and transiting Sun and Mercury were all blessed saving factors.

What was the probable cause? Jupiter rules the health house and fat; Venus rules sugar. Both rule rich foods and particularly sugars. At the beginning of the illness, January 16, the progressed Moon was inconjunct (health aspect) the health house ruler, Jupiter. Sugars had contributed to the cause of the illness. The patient had been given an intravenous supplement of dextrose preceding such examinations and, because of the inability of the body to handle sugars and dextrose, a state of fluctuating coma occurred. In view of the fact that most traumatic experiences herald a lesson of life and that the lesson can be detected through the horoscope, we'll give it a closer inspection.

The Nodes in the natal chart of the Cancer-Capricorn polarity suggest that the native needs to find a balance in family privacy and public expression. The North Node in Capricorn says the native must leave the shell and openly express in order to find emotional peace. As a result of the illness, a new understanding was reached with the mother.

The transiting Nodes were in the same degree, different sign, as progressed Venus, at 17 Taurus-Scorpio. These deserve attention. The position of the Nodes alerts us to an eclipse being not far away. In this instance the eclipse occurred May 4, 1985 at 14 Scorpio, and was in the fifth house of the heart in the patient's chart. Further tests on May 8 revealed the details of a heart condition. The patient was aware there was an abnormality but did not know what it was. Transiting Pluto square natal Neptune describes the condition of the leaky valve.

You are getting the whole story of how these planets joined forces in a particular event which may lead you to believe it is an after-the-fact report only. It is true that the breathing stoppage during the examination was a surprise, but from January 16, 1985 to June 6, 1985, many developments were prepared for in advance through the use and knowledge of complex aspects.

People seldom die when their chart is busy with progressions and transits. Both Neptune and Pluto were heavily energized. Ten months later in the hospital emergency room, feeding tubes were being forced into him and he died resisting these efforts of assistance. He had never lost his appetite; tubes were not necessary. His progressed Moon opposed his natal Moon. The transiting Moon in Scorpio and transiting Jupiter in Pisces formed a grand trine with his natal Ascendant.

The eighth house describes death. Aquarius rules the house cusp and Uranus in the eighth implies the sudden and unexpected. He was taken to the hospital because his heart was malfunctioning. Mars occupies the eighth house in the west side of the chart and rules anger, which could mean assault and struggle. The Sun is also in the eighth house and rules the second, which is said by some to rule one's own death. Neptune in the second could attest that somebody did not know something or did not try to explain, nor did they ask; in other words, confusion. When his throat was attacked it literally frightened him to death. All this is unpleasant, but it does comply with his chart.

Aspects

We will deal only with the most common aspects—the conjunction, the sextile, the square, the trine, the inconjunct, and the opposition.

It seems that all aspects are capable of diversified harmony through their energy. The planets have different energy force from their home station, or the sign they rule, than they do from the sign of detriment (or fall) and/or exaltation.

All planets have more energy from an angular position, less from the succedent houses, and even less from the cadent houses.

Consider whether the planets are applying to the exactness of degree of the aspect or separating from that degree. The applying aspect is more pronounced. Be especially aware fo this if one of the planets is retrograde.

You can select your own keywords indicating wanted or unwanted results and anything in between. Words describe the kind of energy in aspects as favorable and unfavorable, negative and positive, good and evil, good and bad, beneficial and stressful, harmonious and inharmonious, constructive and destructive, benefic and malefic, fortunate and adverse.

Some of the in-between words are neutral, slightly favorable, or slightly unfavorable.

We will use the adjectives favorable and unfavorable with the understanding that any planetary energy can be modified. What may appear unfavorable may actually become a very valuable experience when recognized and when the energy used advantageously. What may at first be considered favorable may expand into unwanted surplus if not used properly.

When dealing with progressions, never more than a two-degree orb is valid. It is suggested that tight orbs be kept when forecasting. When evaluating planetary aspects, be sure to consider whether the planets are approaching the exact degree (applying) or moving farther apart (separating). Pay special attention if one or both are retrograde.

Returning to the chart interpretation, Uranus was retrograde and would go back as far as 15 Sagittarius 00 to form a nearly exact opposition with the natal Moon. This does not mean that the same event will occur; by then, other planets would be forming other aspects, and what was originally an illness could become an event related to sixth-house service.

Conjunction

The conjunction represents the merging of two energy forces. It promotes new beginnings. It is collected power. It brings togetherness. The conjunction may be favorable or unfavorable.

Fitting expressions: "You've got it together." "On target." "Go for it." "Ready, set, go."

42

In the example biwheel chart the natal Moon, transiting Sun, and transiting Mercury are conjunct and collectively rule all the houses from twelve through four. All of the self was thus concentrated in the house of the unconscious or subconscious mind and confinement, which in this instance was a hospital.

Sextile

The sextile is an opportunity that will not manifest without help, and the opportunity can be lost if the individual does nothing to activate it. The sextile is generally favorable but may be neutral.

Fitting expressions: "Keep your hand on the throttle." "Be prepared." "Opportunity may only knock once."

Venus moves more rapidly than Jupiter, but Venus in this example, which was sextile the natal Moon, was progressed and therefore slow. Jupiter was transiting retrograde, which means it would turn direct within four months at the most (the next day in this case) and it was Jupiter that would complete the aspect.

The opportunity from the sextile was two-fold. The native was able to survive. Jupiter from the eighth house gave the opportunity to turn the health around (Jupiter rules the health house). The spiritual attitude (Jupiter) toward the mother was changed. Jupiter rules the natal tenth house, his mother.

Square

The square is accompanied by a crisis, friction, or urgency. It seems sometimes that absolutely nothing would happen until friction makes traction (action). It brings a feeling of urgency and a need to do something. It frequently represents a struggle because friction allows accidents and impulsive action that may require corrective measures.

It may be favorable or unfavorable, depending on the use of the energy, but it is never neutral. Fitting expressions: "Act or react." "Fire only when you see the whites of their eyes." "Too hot to handle."

In the example, the progressed Sun in the tenth reaches for recognition. The Sun was approaching a square to natal Venus in the seventh house, representing the partner. Venus rules the fifth house and the intercepted sign (Taurus) in the eleventh of friends and social activities. The partner can be the tool for favorable publicity, but is also somewhat of a restraint, due to the square.

Let's look at some hypothetical possibilities:

Suppose the progressed Sun were at 21 Aries and natal Venus at 20 Capricorn. The same interpretation would be appropriate, except the action would be in the past. The native would be in the public eye as a result of the partner's love (Venus) and organizational ability (Capricorn). Or the partner could have struggled with the native's success.

Suppose the planets are reversed, with progressed Venus at 20 Aries 43 and the natal Sun at 21 Capricorn 43. The native would be anxious (Aries) and would love to be before the public (Venus in the tenth house). The natal Sun (authority) as partner (seventh house) would try to see to it that it was done, or obstructed, according to what was deserved (Capricorn), be it good publicity or bad.

Suppose these planets were reversed by degree, with Venus progressed to 21 Aries 43 and the natal Sun at 20 Capricorn 43. The native would have been financially successful or unsuccessful, or hurt through love because of the partner.

Trine

Luck, abundance, ease, fortune, and expansion describe the trine aspect. The trine has both planets in the same element unless very near a sign cusp; then it may be an out-of-sign aspect. The ease factor can manifest as neglect and can eliminate success and ambition. It can bring an abundance of the unwanted (negative or unfortunate).

Fitting expressions: "Guardian angel." "From out of nowhere." "A gift of God." "Too much of anything is enough."

In the example, the unexpected (Uranus) occurred when one of the physicians ordered more tests as the patient was getting ready to leave the hospital.

Now let us suppose these planets were reversed with Uranus in the twelfth house and the Sun in the eighth and that previous developments had brought the same circumstances. The native's freedom (Uranus) would have been restricted (twelfth house) because the Sun in the eighth house would have indicated surgery with good results. There might have even been a miracle healing "as a gift of God."

Inconjunct

The inconjunct implies a dilemma or a change due to circumstances out of the native's control. It presents a situation to which the native can hopefully react to constructively. There are six signs between one planet and the other. The inconjunct is always present in health charts. In the other direction, the planets are eight signs apart; this is the regenerative aspect.

Organic conditions are defined by the six-signs aspect, and accidents by the eight-signs aspect. Fitting expressions: "Born again." "Swimming upstream." "One day at a time." "Serve or be served." "Marching to a different drummer."

In the example, there are six signs from progressed Neptune to transiting Neptune (health angle). Neptune indicates toxins in the body and mysterious health problems. Counting the other direction, or eight signs, the aspect indicates that a regeneration of attitude toward values could assist the improvement in health through mental attitude.

Opposition

The opposition is like one of the laws of nature: "opposites attract." It represents separation, cooperation, and completion and is supplementary. Awareness is another applicable interpretation for the opposition.

The opposition of the Sun and Moon has a Full Moon effect. The Sun reflects light on the Moon and light is supplied during the dark hours. There are always two people, things, events, or attitudes involved. The separation provides awareness of the need to cooperate in order to gain the benefits of needed qualities from the opposite sign. There is no competition without an opponent. You don't play in the tournament if you don't sign up.

In interpreting the opposition it may be helpful to remember that the seventh house, which is opposition the first, rules both marriage and divorce. Therefore, the opposition can be both favorable and unfavorable. Fitting expressions: "It takes two to tango." "Wedded bliss." "If you can't lick 'em, join 'em."

In the example there are four oppositions. The first is transiting Neptune opposition natal and progressed Pluto. Both Pluto and Neptune are mysterious. Pluto can unveil and Neptune dissolves. Notice that transiting Neptune is at a later minute than natal Pluto, meaning the opposition was exact earlier that day. Neptune was retrograde and the ephemeris shows the aspect will be exact twice more. Health conditions heretofore either unknown or ignored, maybe some of both, were unveiled and some of the problems were dissolved when Neptune formed the exact aspect the first time.

Another opposition is of the second-eighth house polarity and relates to values, both material and spiritual. It is perfectly natural for anyone to scrutinize values very closely upon the realization that life is a fine line from death.

When the transiting Moon opposed Neptune the patient was temporarily out of touch with reality due to the medication received at the hospital.

It has long been known that transiting Neptune opposition, conjunction, or square the natal Moon, and to a lesser extent the Moon transiting opposition, conjunction, or square natal Neptune, can have an intoxicating impression. Alcoholics drink more under these transits and sugar has the same effect on those who are allergic to it. It is becoming more widely accepted that it is the sugar that is the addiction. Sugar is as damaging to the body as alcohol and destroys the same organs.

The third set of oppositions is a fifth-eleventh house polarity. The eleventh house rules friends, clubs, and social activities, and the fifth house rules children, pleasures, and the heart. After the interruption in breathing during the strobe test, the next step was to examine the heart. The reason the patient would become short of breath while walking was promptly revealed.

It has been found that interceptions sometimes provide protection. The individual is protected from that which is "shut out"; the fifth and eleventh houses are intercepted, protecting from heart failure.

Before going on to the fourth opposition let us blend the last two sets of oppositions, which formed a fixed grand cross. Anyone experiencing more than two aspects to natal or progressed planets in fixed signs should treat the heart with respect and particularly if one of the planets is in the fifth house, rules the fifth house, or is the Sun or Mars. Here we have the transiting co-ruler of the fifth in the intercepted sign in the fifth.

The Moon will quickly move out of orb, but be mindful that it will return to Aquarius every twenty-eight days. The slow motion of Pluto in aspect to natal and progressed planets can be lengthy, and sets the stage set for several months or years. After transiting Pluto resume direct motion and was applying to an exact aspect to Mercury and Neptune at three degrees, any transit of 3 Aquarius could indicate significant action of some kind.

The sixth and twelfth house oppositions were in water and earth signs and sextile transiting Pluto and progressed Venus. Transiting Neptune, which was sextile transiting Pluto, was also trine progressed Mercury, and progressed Mercury was just past the exact sextile to natal Pluto. When Mercury was well within orb to natal Pluto the native made a drastic dietary change which proved to be very satisfactory. Neptune transiting the sixth house of food, coming to a trine with progressed Mercury, provided Neptunian instinct as to what the body needed. There is that trine angel again.

Mercury in Taurus suggests rest and relaxation. The placement in the eleventh house in the intercepted sign suggests that social exchange would be beneficial, but it would be unwise to hold office in an organization or club because of the Mercury tie-in to the fixed grand cross.

Transiting Pluto was trine natal and progressed Pluto. The co-ruler of the heart, in this chart, in transit and in aspect to the same planet in the natal chart in the twelfth house implies that the native did self-damage (self-undoing) in the past (probably eating and drinking (Pluto in Cancer).

Note the progressed Moon. It had been within orb to one or more of the opposition planets since the onset of the illness on January 16. That orb was widening in June, meaning the crisis was over. It had progressed to the point of a yod with progressed Mercury and natal Pluto.

Let's examine a yod more closely using the example given. Progressed Mercury and natal and progressed Pluto were sextile, allowing an opportunity. The progressed Moon was six signs from progressed Mercury and eight signs from both natal and progressed Pluto. The sixth house count has the option of health or service. The eighth house count has the option of change. The eighth house also rules debts and creditors.

Anyone operating under a yod may do well to examine the past and find what is owed to someone else. It could be a karmic debt and not a material one. The two inconjuncts in a yod are supplemented by the sextile of opportunity delivering the difficult events and changes that come with an out-of-your-control inconjunct but with a built-in escape hatch through the sextile where gains can be made and lessons can be learned. Perhaps this is why the yod is called the finger of God.

The last opposition was transiting Uranus opposition the natal Moon. This is another sixth-twelfth house polarity. Notice that Uranus was in the sign of abundance, Sagittarius, and that the health house is ruled by Jupiter, which is afflicted in the natal chart by a square from Saturn in the first house. The Moon rules the Ascendant.

As can be seen, many of the aspects pointed to illness and confinement. When a number of aspects occur at the same time, the use of keywords will point to the major activity or attitude being experienced at the time.

Semioctile

It may well be that everyone reading this book is fully aware of the energy of the minor aspect called the semioctile, but my knowledge was vague until it was brought to my attention. The semioctile is 22°30′ or half of a semisquare. In her book *Minor Aspects*, Emma Belle Donath wrote, "There is reason to believe that the semioctile aspect is particularly involved with health concerns which would certainly follow in the wake of excellent medical research done by Reinhold Ebertin and his associates." She added: "The separating aspect means 'speed up' and the applying energy means 'slow down.'"

Progressed and transiting aspects to the date of the illness, June 6, 1985, are listed below. In the natal chart the semioctile may promote a struggle to stay well when ill or a struggle to appear ill for convenience.

- Natal Pluto at 2 Cancer 40 semioctile natal Saturn at 25 Cancer 55 (45′ orb)
- Natal Mercury at 19 Capricorn 53 semioctile natal Sun at 12 Aquarius 26 (3′ orb). He was overly cautious concerning health issues, but too late in life to save damaged organs.

- Natal Chiron at 23 Pisces 23 semioctile progressed Venus at 16 Aries 46 (53' orb). Chiron is frequently prominent in illness. Venus represents the sugar injections.
- Progressed Chiron at 27 Pisces 16 semioctile progressed Sun 20 Aries 43 (57' orb). Provides a strong warning with regard to alcohol abuse.
- Progressed Mars at 11 Aries 57 semioctile progressed Mercury at 3 Taurus 50 (32' orb). Much effort was directed toward nutrition.

The following three semioctile aspects show a link between Chiron, Pluto, and Saturn:

- Natal Saturn at 25 Cancer 55 semioctile progressed Pluto at 2 Cancer 27 (58' orb). Progressed Pluto had returned to its exact natal position and was semioctile natal Saturn, which represented karma with other people.
- Natal Pluto at 2 Cancer 40 semioctile transiting Chiron at 9 Gemini 25 (45'). This aspect seemed to prepare for the realization of impending death.
- Transiting Chiron at 9 Gemini 25 semioctile transiting North Node at 16 Taurus 51 (4' orb). The North Node closes karma. Note: Chiron is at the midpoint of the transiting North Node and natal Pluto, and natal Pluto is at the midpoint of transiting Chiron and natal Saturn which links three different semioctile aspects.
- Transiting Saturn at 23 Scorpio 15 semioctile transiting Uranus at 16 Sagittarius (5' orb). Shows the things that were happening at the moment, a life and death emergency; calcium was forming in the heart valves.

Natal chart with progressions and transits to the date of the death event, March 28, 1986 are listed below. To begin, note that the Chiron-Pluto-Saturn aspect referenced above was still in effect ten months later.

- Natal Midheaven at 19 Pisces 31 semioctile progressed

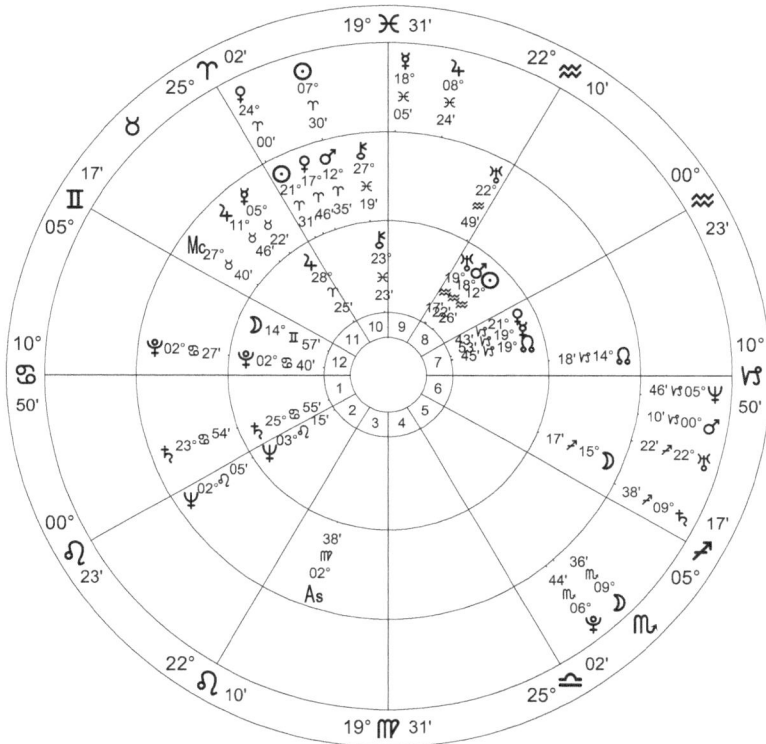

Jim Garrett. Inner wheel, natal chart; middle wheel, progressed, March 28, 1986; outer wheel, transits, March 28, 1986, 5:50 am

    Mars at 12 Aries 35. Of all the patients at the hospital, he was in the center of attention.
- Progressed North Node at 14 Capricorn 18 semioctile transiting Uranus at 22 Sagittarius 22. Everyone was surprised by his death. In fact, I expected him to live for two more weeks. But he knew.

Chiron is frequently involved in death charts (see chart above for the date and time of Jim's death):

- Transiting Chiron at 10 Gemini 15 trine natal Sun at 12 Aquarius 26.
- Transiting Uranus at 22 Sagittarius 22 sextile progressed Uranus at 22 Aquarius 49.
- Natal Chiron at 23 Pisces 23 square transiting Uranus at 22 Sagittarius 22.

At death, transiting Chiron was closely trine natal Sun, and transiting Uranus was sextile progressed Uranus and closely square natal Chiron.

Chapter 4

Appetite Versus Addiction

Some people insist that when there is a craving for a food it means the body needs that food. This makes as much sense as saying that when an alcoholic craves another drink, the body is in need of it.

Well, guess what? This kind of thinking is the link to one of America's greatest agonies—allergies. Most people are shocked when they eventually discover that the very food they think is helpful to them is the exact food to which they are allergic. This is an extremely difficult point to prove because the body does feel better for a few minutes after partaking of the allergen, just as an alcoholic feels better for a few minutes after having another drink. So what is the answer? Absolute honesty and abstinence must be practiced. If it is an allergen to you, it is a 100 percent no-no!

I was born with sensitive skin and was not allowed to attend school at ages six and seven. My skin looked so bad from my allergies that some people thought I had "something that was catching," and I also could not hold a pencil to participate in written assignments. A similar major outbreak occurred at age fourteen and again at age twenty when twice the limit of x-ray treatment was administered. A very dramatic event was experienced with cortisone treatment when it was first released to the medical profession. That was during my first Saturn return. The lesson I was to learn, evidently, was that the sulfur, which was always a part of any medication for eczema in those days, was the element to which I was most highly allergic. Saturn rules both skin and sulfur.

Shortly after that, I was fortunate enough to experience hypnotherapy and was taught self-hypnosis. It was through a careful search of the subconscious that the cause was identified. During the past forty-two years of blessed relief and freedom from allergy, there have been no outbreaks beyond warning signals that have prompted a review of cause and consequential recovery. The disappointment is that so very few people believe we can control our allergies. They apparently just want to stop with the allergen. We cannot stop there. We must go back to the emotion that permits the allergen to take over.

There are three stages to an allergic manifestation:

1. The gene must be inherited.

2. There must be an emotional condition to permit the invasion. (The emotional condition must be faced and dealt with. The cure dwells there.)

3. The allergen must be present. However, even if it is present it cannot invade if we emotionally stabilize against it. Physical exposure to allergens can usually be managed in tolerance and with common sense.

So you ask, "What has this to do with appetite and addiction?" There certainly are occasions where our appetite and cravings are valid. The difference is that when the need is satisfied, the craving goes away until the body needs that element again. However, a constant craving usually is for that to which we are allergic. Immediately we recognize the close relationship to addiction. Addictions often connect with energy level and/or emotional needs.

Sweets are the earliest exposure we have to a potential addiction; one of the major ingredients of milk from any animal source is lactose, a form of sugar. When a baby is weaned, it is not weaned from the sweet taste; it is only weaned from the method of taking the sweet. All too frequently the baby ends up transferring the need for the sweet taste to cookies and candy. The milk, which represents the necessary protein supply, is then dropped. Substitute milk formula may contain dehydrated animal milk and some form of sweetener or soybean base that supplies vegetable protein. Soybean is a carbohydrate that immediately converts into sugar and instant energy and is much higher in caloric content than animal milk with its natural fat, most of which has been removed from the dried milk base.

Hopefully, some of this information will be helpful in feeding a baby who is overweight or experiencing allergies. The baby's allergies might also be due to neglect, an overly protective environment, abuse from someone or some inner nature that the child cannot yet express. An astrological reading can be valuable to both child and parents in such an instance.

Look for sugar addictions to be astrologically associated with Venus, Libra, Taurus, and Pisces. The ruler of the eleventh house (returned love) is afflicted in some way in every chart I have seen of a known diabetic.

A client called me about a child who had been rushed to the hospital for what was thought to be a seizure. A horary chart was examined and the frantic grandmother was advised not to be concerned. The child was being held too tightly and not allowed sufficient freedom. If such control continued, the child would most likely develop asthma, but it was not a seizure.

She sent a note with her check thanking me for the comments and advised that, surprisingly, her daughter had heard her out and was pleased to report that the child had not had a seizure but was holding his breath. This brings us to one of the emotional allergies—asthma, a struggle for freedom. Astrologically, look for it under Jupiter, Sagittarius, Uranus, and Aquarius.

Any allergy of the respiratory system relates to being denied the privilege of communication, or the self-punishment of regretting some expression. With respect to food, the offenders could well be vegetables that grow on vines. Seafood, especially shellfish, are also disturbing to subjects inclined to respiratory disorders.

Allergies related to the head, nasal cavity, eyes, headaches, etc., associate with the need to express the "I am." The individual might be living too completely in someone else's shadow or might be denying self a priority life. Honesty to one's self can cure the allergy, even if only by continuing life with the one simple change: "Admit that it is not as important to be different as it is to be what you are expected to be."

The other choice is to develop the courage to make some changes. Headaches point to self-concern and people may be sympathetic but can get bored by it. Headaches are tough to deal with because they are extremely difficult to forget when they're your own. The food allergies are most likely to be milk or grain foods such as wheat. Both are congestive. Would milk relate to the infant's need to grow and become independent? And would the grains, being the staff of life, relate to the need for the security of a calm, substantial home life?

Allergies of the skin are exactly what the following metaphor implies: the individual is breaking out to be different. The choice is break out or break down. Skin eruptions promote becoming a social outcast; they leave the appearance of being unclean. The most common allergen to skin reactions is acid foods, including various meats that break down into acids during the digestion process. Remember, it is said that fats make acne, and pork is credited with fever blisters on the lips.

We continue to transfer the sweet taste all through life. People who quit smoking go directly to gum, candy or other sweets (carbo-junk). Somewhere along the way when we meet with an emotional crisis or loneliness, we pamper ourselves with sweets.

56

When carbohydrates, cakes, candy, cookies, or Cokes (notice all the C's) don't give satisfaction, we then transfer our sweet tooth to alcohol, which is approximately the same percentage of sugar as its alcohol content because the sugar converts to alcohol in the distillation process just as sugar converts to alcohol (energy) inside the body. Alcohol, being already converted, denies the liver that service, and the liver begins to become inactive. If threatened long enough, the liver hardens—cirrhosis.

Chocolate is an appetite and, like coffee, it contains caffeine, which is also an addiction. Because neither tastes good to the untrained palate, people have to learn to develop a taste for coffee and chocolate; sugar makes it easy. We get quickly digested energy from sweets, but the trouble is that refined sugar does not supply energy. It just multiplies into cells that stay in the body and add weight. Energy to use up these cells has to come from other more wholesome foods. Caffeine has few calories but provides high energy because it is a stimulant. Chocolate thus has two vices—more caffeine than coffee and major sweeteners. Caffeine is not handled well by the liver, which is pushed to support sufficient energy to burn off the excessive sweet calories. Caffeine does have some advantages; the problem is in knowing when we are getting hooked into an addiction for energy rather than getting it from protein (which actually provides strength) and carbohydrates.

We might consider the taste for nicotine. We don't actually eat tobacco but half a century ago practically every family had more than one male who chewed tobacco or women who dipped snuff (powdered tobacco). One of the sneak tricks when I was a child was to dip sugar and cocoa (the caffeine in chocolate). There's that sugar word again! Nicotine is a stimulant that causes the blood to flow. When I quit smoking, I did it by taking an occasional small portion of a niacin (nicotinic acid or Vitamin-B) tablet because it gave me a smaller substitute rush of circulation. If you try it, please be careful to not overdo. Do not take more than a tablet a day for three or four days; use it for crisis moments only.

Another appetite is for salt, which can also become an addiction. The emotional base for craving salt is the desire to flush feelings out of life. The harboring of emotions manifests into fluid retention. Most people who retain fluids excessively will maintain that they use little or no salt. This is probably true in the sense that they do not use a salt shaker. Salt is noted as sodium on prepared food cartons and carbonated drink cans. Soda is short for sodium; table salt is sodium chloride. Anyone who holds excessive fluids should make an assertive effort to let go (and let God) of something or someone and live in the present, not the past, with an eye toward the future.

A great part of the medical profession does not believe that what we eat has anything to do with our health. It puzzles me as to why these same practitioners write great books on prescriptions for pills to be put into the body by the same process by which we eat. On the other hand, it was not until recently that few, if any, schools of medicine required even a single class on nutrition. The truth is medical doctors know less about food than some of us know about medicine. So if you want to know something about what you should eat, don't ask a doctor.

The natal horoscope displays everything in our lives, even the way we eat. Everyone has an appetite suitable in some way to the characteristics of the birth chart. Zodiacal sign traits can also be applied to the Sun sign, Moon sign, and rising sign (the Ascendant) and to the sixth house of the natal chart; these rule food preparation and health. Any planet in the first house or conjunct the natal Sun also impresses the appetite.

These points describe the taste preferences, the habits of consumption and how the body reacts to the food consumed. For example, a person with a Taurus Sun may like the favorite Taurus sign foods. If he has the Moon in Aries, he might eat fast or might like spicy Aries sign foods. Let's give him a Virgo Ascendant, which would indicate his full appreciation of vegetables. The "hungries" don't necessarily come on schedule, which is in keeping with Aquarius on the sixth house cusp. The need for food is governed by the fourth house, which rules the stomach. That sign is Sagittarius and the requirement is massive.

This is a real person and he eats like this: He prefers hamburger to beef steak. He does like spicy food and eats fast. The Virgo Ascendant instills that he eat healthy foods, and as he says, "As long as there is enough of it." This statement is also upheld by the Sun in the ninth house, Sagittarius's natural place. Aquarius has no schedule; it operates on priorities of free will. In this example, the stomach is ruled by Sagittarius; when it is empty it must have *something.*

Chapter 5

Food and Alcohol

Whiskey and bourbon drinkers are of two kinds: They tend to have a need to reflect a tough image or they are exceptionally well-dressed and want peers to think they can control themselves and any situation.

Bourbon is French whiskey and is made from the malt of corn or rye. Malt is a grain that has been sprouted in water, and is then distilled and aged in charred oak containers. Anyone who is known to be allergic to corn or rye should avoid bourbon. Whiskey is made form corn, barley, or wheat that has been fermented, distilled, and aged. It should be avoided by those who are allergic to corn, barley, or wheat.

People who drink scotch are usually a little knowledgeable in nutrition and mix it with water only, knowing there is less chance for a hangover. Scotch promotes a controlled relaxation, normally leaving nothing to regret tomorrow from yesterday's events.

Scotch is rye whiskey, a specialty of Scotland, and is made by the same process as whiskey. Rye is rated low as an allergen and is safe for most people, but the rare person who is allergic to rye should avoid scotch. Any kind of alcohol can be readily overdone and become addictive.

Many who drink vodka think nobody knows they are drinking, but they forget that drinking sends one to the restroom, which requires a walk from the chair or bar stool. Vodka doesn't smell, but it shows in the gait.

Vodka is made from fermented, distilled rye or wheat that has not been aged. Some vodka is made from potatoes and is of Russian origin. Vodka should be avoided by anyone allergic to rye, wheat, or potatoes.

Rum belongs more to the occasional party drinker who decides to have a fun night out. Rum is sweet and potent and generally is mixed with fruit juice, which sweetens it even more. The symbology in these drinks is to sweeten life for a few hours. It is hard to get by an evening of rum without a hangover. The liver gets confused; the rum is already alcohol, but the fruit or juice needs to be converted.

Rum is manufactured for the American market primarily on tropical islands, such as in the Caribbean. It is made from cane molasses. Molasses is similar to sugar cane but much higher in iron. Alcohol tends to imbalance iron with copper by sending excessive copper to the brain and escalating iron in the blood stream, and rum will accentuate that process. Anyone with such an imbalance of iron and copper should avoid rum.

Gin is another party drink more frequently mixed with a fizz or carbonated drink of some kind It is usually flavored with fruit rather than mixed with juice. Here is the party animal who seeks fun, not oblivion.

Gin is made from juniper berries and distilled. Juniper berries can be toxic to the body, especially to the kidneys even though they are one of the remedies for kidney disorders. Tolerance is the keyword. Excess consumption of gin or juniper berries can bring irreparable damage to the kidneys.

Tequila makes pretty drinks with a flair. These drinks add drama to a party and call attention to the drinker. Tequila is Mexican, and accentuates spicy food, which can balance it better than less bold mixtures.

Tequila, a distilled liquor that is usually unaged, is made from the fermented juice of the Mexican agave (tequila cactus) plant. This beverage was developed soon after the Spaniards introduced distillation to Mexico. Upon maturity, the pineapple-like agave plant's base fills with a sweet sap. This juice is fermented and then distilled twice to achieve the desired purity.

Tequila is mixed with lime juice and an orange-flavored liqueur to make a Margarita, which is served in a glass rimmed with salt. Traditional tequila drinkers usually prefer it unmixed, accompanied by salt and a lime slice. The drinker takes salt, tequila, and lime in rapid succession, thus combining all the flavors. Mescal, a similar distilled beverage, is less expensive and stronger in flavor. It is made from an agave plant that grows wild in the Oaxaca region of Mexico.

Sake is an Oriental wine made from rice. It has the wallop of strong whiskey, and it seems to me that Americans drink it to show off their drinking ability. My opinion is that it must be had on a stomach full of tofu or other soy bean base. Sake goes wild on meat protein such as beef or pork.

Wine falls in two categories, dry and sweet. Wine drinkers are lovers. Those who prefer dry wine tend to drink little or nothing else. Those who prefer sweet wine might drink little or nothing else except on romantic occasions or they might have a tropical mix once in a while at a bar or dinner with a group. Men are more likely to choose the dry red wines, and ladies go for white or rose, sweeter wines of the more floral aroma.

Wine enjoys the longest history of any of the alcoholic beverages. It obviously was a discovery, not an invention. Grapes quench thirst, and juice loads in a goat skin much lighter than whole grapes. Grapes are seasonal and ferment before the next crop. Wine is that simple to make but the process can be escalated by adding yeast to expedite fermentation. Not all wine contains sulfites. Read the label. Sulfites cause headaches in most people.

Wine can be beneficial. Approximately three ounces of red wine daily can be very good for a weak heart condition. But one does not need to resort to the addictive risk or expense of wine for this benefit. Grape juice does the same thing. The redder, the better.

Champagne is, as my late husband often said, recycled wine. Champagne is twice distilled, which gives the sparkle and fizz. Fizz automatically prompts a party atmosphere. However, if all the yeast has not escaped from champagne, a headache can follow. Champagne derives its name from a region in France.

Brandy is a heavy wine or fruited whiskey. It has a high content of alcohol, is seldom made from anything other than fruit and has little or no water content. Brandy is a good cough syrup, used in tolerance, but it could upset the stomach.

Beer and ale drinkers are the laughers. The drink fizzes and buzzes and so do the consumers. Beer and ale people are seldom mournful and sympathy seeking. The hops may put some of them to sleep rather quickly, but the others eat, drink ,and make merry until they wind down and then go to bed.

The hop plant is a climbing vine and a member of the mulberry family. The dried cones of the female flowers quickly lend themselves to fermentation, which can result in intoxication. Anyone who is allergic to penicillin might have a problem drinking beer. Beer can be brewed from various plant products but most beer in the United States is brewed from corn or rice. An occasional beer or ale will aid in flushing the kidney and urinary bladder just as yeast tablets flush septic tanks. To do the same thing without beer, drink more water than usual for a few hours and then put your buttocks on a couch, your feet over the top of the couch, and your shoulders on the floor and hold that position for about fifteen or twenty minutes.

Chapter 6

Carbonated and Fruit Beverages

The first assignment of the day for at least one office employee is to make coffee and have it ready for the rest of the crew when they arrive. Somewhere there is likely to be a ten-gallon water jug supplied for a fee by a commercial distributor. Industries, office complexes, schools, and other locations have vending machines with assorted drinks available.

You are driving behind a pickup truck, possibly a construction worker, and you see a ten-gallon thermos container or a large chest cooler. It might contain anything from plain water to beer. In another car is a man dressed in a business suit. He probably has some level of office equipment with him—telephone, receipt pad, calculator or laptop. He also has a thirty-two ounce container of some kind of drink he picked up at a coffee place or when he bought gas. Trudging along the sidewalk is a young woman in walking shoes to support her swollen ankles, and she is caressing a quart-sized container with a tall sucking tube so she hardly has to bend her neck to prevent thirst as she replaces all the damaging chemistry her body tried desperately to remove during the night. Most of these people will be from twenty to 150 pounds overweight.

"But I drink only diet drinks," someone exclaims. What's wrong here? Chemical content! Let's bump coffee first. All-day coffee drinkers are less likely to be overweight because coffee has caffeine, an energizer that works off everything else except high caffeine soda drinks that the coffee drinker may switch to in the afternoon. The caffeine addiction must be satisfied, but sodium stays thirsty and causes the body to retain fluids. At least one-third of the twenty to 150 pounds mentioned in the above paragraph is likely to be fluid.

The chemistry in diet drinks promotes fluid retention, destroys natural protection against high blood pressure and usually contains a chemical that depresses the brain. Food then becomes an unlabeled restaurant killer or a diet preparation loaded with sodium, fully dedicated to destroying valuable body strength. That much sodium (salt) stimulates thirst.

Many foods and drinks contain aspartame, also known as NutraSweet or Equal. It contains aspartic acid (aspartame), which inhibits the function of the thymus gland (immune system support); phenylalanine, which should never be consumed by anyone who has anxiety attacks; and methanol, which converts to formaldehyde and formic acid, both of which have an adverse effect on the thymus gland. Aspartame is a dangerous additive *(Prescriptions for Nutritional Healing*, p. 133, James F. and Phyllis A. Balch, Avery Publishing Group, 1990).

All of the above increase the likelihood of heart problems, diabetes, and cancer, the three leading causes of death in the United States. They even promote accidents, next high on the list. We all do die of something, but there is more quality in life for one who goes healthy.

If you are absolutely compelled to drink carbonated drinks, the non-diet variety is far better for you. Yes, they have calories. They also give you energy that you feel like using instead of filling you with another half gallon of liquid (four pounds) that you have to carry with you every step. If you really need to diet, do it right. Eat.

Water, very weak tea or diluted juice is better fluid than anything with carbonation.

Fruit juice can be a treat, but to some it is a threat. It is easy enough to enjoy a cup full of grapes in which you get 120 to 140 calories, fiber, and liquid. It would take four to five cups of grapes to render a cup of juice that would contain little or no fiber and more than 500 calories. So, energy-wise, a 1:1 cup of juice and a 3:1 cup of water makes for a vital drink. Any bottled juice drink should be closely examined for sugar and additive content, which should absolutely avoided. Natural (nature) is best!

Be aware that canned or bottled fruit juice often has additives you can do without. Read the label. Frozen is a more wholesome choice, but fresh whole fruit is best. It takes more effort to eat it, but chances are you need exercise, so a trip to the trash can to throw away the skin and seeds is helpful and a trip to the bathroom to wash your hands won't hurt either. Americans spend millions for exercise every year and you can get it free just by getting off the couch and eating fresh fruit!

Chapter 7

Food Additives and Enhancers

A small percentage of people are sensitive to monosodium glutamate. This white crystalline powder is a salt of glutamic acid that occurs naturally in sugar beets, soybeans, and seaweed. It can also be manufactured synthetically. Perhaps it is best to bear in mind that salt is a salt, even if it is made of sugar. In short, if you need to be alert to salt or sugar, beware of MSG.

Salt is added to food for taste or as a preservative. Sodium nitrate, a chemical form of salt, is added as a preservative to cure meat, bacon, ham, sausage, lunch meat, and other foods. It is known to cause health problems. Too many people who think they use no salt are taking in excessive amounts through habitual consumption of preserved foods. Regular table salt, vinegar, and sugar are also some of the preservatives often added.

The below list of herbs and spices might be helpful in reducing the use of salt or sugar. Only a few suggested uses are included. They enhance taste and can be healing agents.

Helpful Herbs and Spices

Ailment	Herb/Spice	Suggested Use
Arthritis	Cayenne pepper garlic	Pasta, vegies
Anemia	Cayenne pepper, garlic, parsley	Pasta, vegies
Asthma	Anise, licorice, sage garlic, ginger, onion, rosemary, thyme	Drinks, poultry, vegies
Blood purifier	Dandelion	Salads with greens
Bronchitis	Anise, licorice, horseradish, garlic, ginger, thyme	Drinks, meats, vegies
Circulation	Cayenne pepper, ginger, cinnamon	Meat, fruit, vegies
Colds	Cayenne pepper, ginger, onion, sage, marjoram, saffron, parsley, rosemary	Soup, vegies
Colic	Anise, bay, ginger, caraway, cinnamon, dill, cumin, fennel, marjoram, cardamon, oregano, savory, rosemary, spearmint	Soup, tea
Constipation	Fennel, ginger, pepper	Fiber
Cough	Anise, horseradish, licorice, onion, thyme, marjoram, oregano	Drinks, soup, vegies
Cramps	Fennel, ginger	Meat, soup, tea

70

Ailment	Herb/Spice	Suggested Use
Diabetes	Dandelion, fennel	Tea, soup, salad
Diarrhea	Cinnamon, ginger, pepper	Soup, tea
Dizziness	Dandelion, marjoram	As desired
Fever	Cayenne pepper, fennel, ginger, parsley, thyme, tarragon	As desired
Flatulence	Allspice, anise, bay leaf, sage, clove, cardamon, cumin, marjoram, garlic, dandelion, fennel	Vegies
Gallstones	Horseradish, Tarragon, parsley	As desired
Headache	Marjoram, oregano, rosemary, thyme	Pasta
Hysteria	Bay leaf, caraway, celery	As desired
Indigestion	Anise, bay leaf, sage, caraway, dandelion, cayenne pepper, cardamon, fennel, thyme, marjoram, rosemary, garlic	Vegies, meat
Insomnia	Anise, onion	Drink, sandwich
Kidney/bladder	Parsley, tarragon	Tea, salad
Kidney/liver	Dandelion, sage	As desired
Nausea	Clove, ginger, pepper, oregano, spearmint	As desired

Ailment	Herb/Spice	Suggested Use
Nervousness	Bay leaf, celery, rosemary, sage	Soup, salad, vegies
Obesity	Dandelion, fennel, garlic	As desired
Rheumatism	Basil, celery, chicory, fennel, garlic, Oregano, horseradish	Meat, vegies
Sinus	Garlic	As desired
Skin problems	Dandelion, parsley	Tea
Sore throat	Ginger, onion, oregano	As desired
Toothache	Cloves	Chew
Stomach upset	Fennel, oregano, Chicory	As desired
Urinary infection	Horseradish	Sparingly

A few leaves of dandelion is an excellent addition to salad. No insecticide!

Horseradish is excellent for colds, sinus, kidney. Use no more than one-half teaspoon per day and for no more than a week. Wait at least one week to use again.